WHAT'S INSIDE ME?

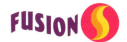

My BRAIN

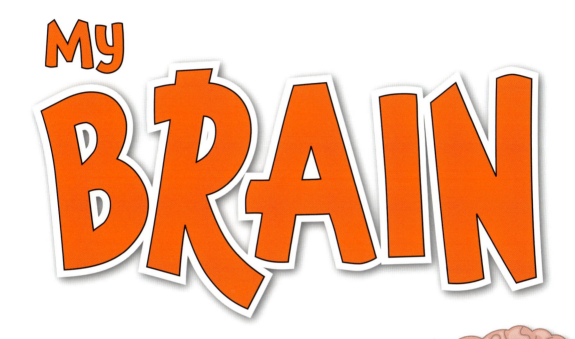

by Sloane Hughes

BEARPORT
PUBLISHING

Minneapolis, Minnesota

Credits: Cover, all background, © Piotr Urakau/Shutterstock; cover, 7, 23 © BlueRingMedia/Shutterstock; cover, 4, 10, 14, 16, 21–22 brain illustration © Shutterstock; 4 Sergey Novikov/Shutterstock; 5 Samuel Borges Photography/Shutterstock; 6 (brain) r.classen/Shutterstock; 6 (fist) Lipik Stock Media/Shutterstock; 9 VikiVector/Shutterstock; 10 Taleseedum/Shutterstock; Anna Kraynova/Shutterstock; 12 MicroOne/Shutterstock; 13 Monkey Business Images/Shutterstock; 14–15 (lightning) Freud/Shutterstock; 15 Magic mine/Shutterstock; 16 Romanova Natali/Shutterstock; 17 antoniodiaz/Shutterstock; 18 Sergey Novikov/Shutterstock; 19 marilyn barbone/Shutterstock; 20 Beatriz Gascon J/ Shutterstock; 21 fizkes/Shutterstock;

President: Jen Jenson
Director of Product Development: Spencer Brinker
Senior Editor: Allison Juda
Associate Editor: Charly Haley
Designer: Oscar Norman

Library of Congress Cataloging-in-Publication Data

Names: Hughes, Sloane, author.
Title: My brain / by Sloane Hughes.
Description: Fusion books. | Minneapolis, Minnesota : Bearport Publishing
    Company, [2022] | Series: What's inside me? | Includes index.
Identifiers: LCCN 2021039154 (print) | LCCN 2021039155 (ebook) | ISBN
    9781636914411 (library binding) | ISBN 9781636914480 (paperback) | ISBN
    9781636914558 (ebook)
Subjects: LCSH: Brain--Juvenile literature.
Classification: LCC QP376 .H856 2022 (print) | LCC QP376 (ebook) | DDC
    612.8/2--dc23
LC record available at https://lccn.loc.gov/2021039154
LC ebook record available at https://lccn.loc.gov/2021039155

Copyright © 2022 Bearport Publishing Company. All rights reserved. No part of this publication may be reproduced in whole or in part, stored in any retrieval system, or transmitted in any form or by any means, electronic, mechanical, photocopying, recording, or otherwise, without written permission from the publisher.

For more information, write to Bearport Publishing, 5357 Penn Avenue South, Minneapolis, MN 55419. Printed in the United States of America.

CONTENTS

The Inside Scoop 4
A Job to Do 6
What's in Your Head? 8
Talented Twins 10
Taking It All In 12
Brain Buddies........................14
A New Path 16
Taking Care of You! 18
A Good Night's Rest 20
Your Busy Body....................22
Glossary.................................24
Index 24

THE INSIDE SCOOP

Your body is a super machine that keeps you moving, learning, and having fun. But how does it work? The secret is inside!

You'll think I'm super cool!

When you open a book, your brain lets you read the words and see the pictures. It even helps you turn the page! Let's learn more about the brain.

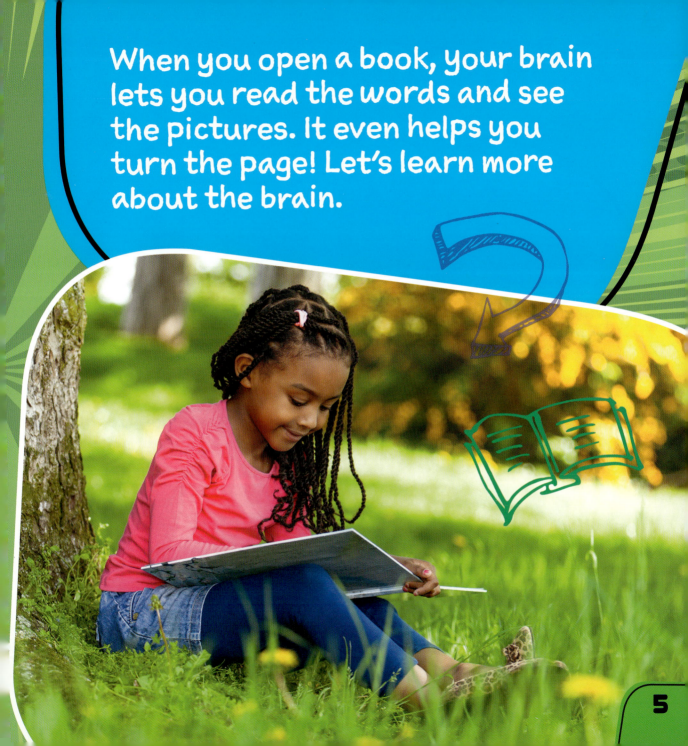

A JOB TO DO

Your brain is hard at work in your head. Bones around your brain keep it safe so it can take care of everything else.

An adult's brain is about the size of two fists put together.

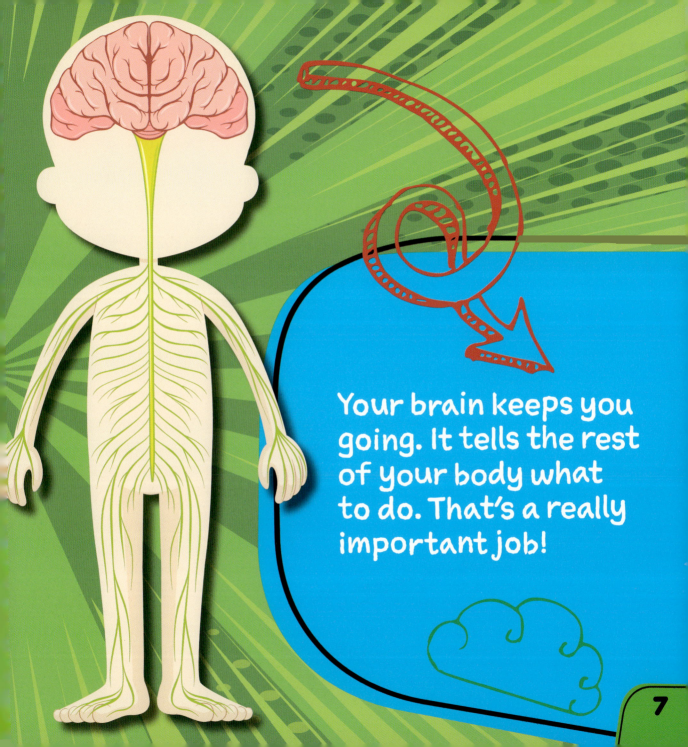

WHAT'S IN YOUR HEAD?

There are three parts of your brain. The largest is the cerebrum (suh-REE-bruhm). The cerebellum (ser-uh-BEL-uhm) is a smaller part at the back. And the brain stem comes out of the bottom of your brain.

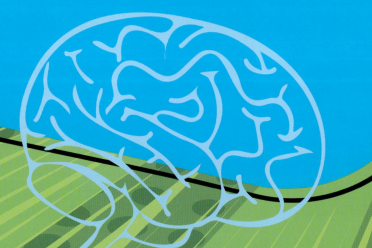

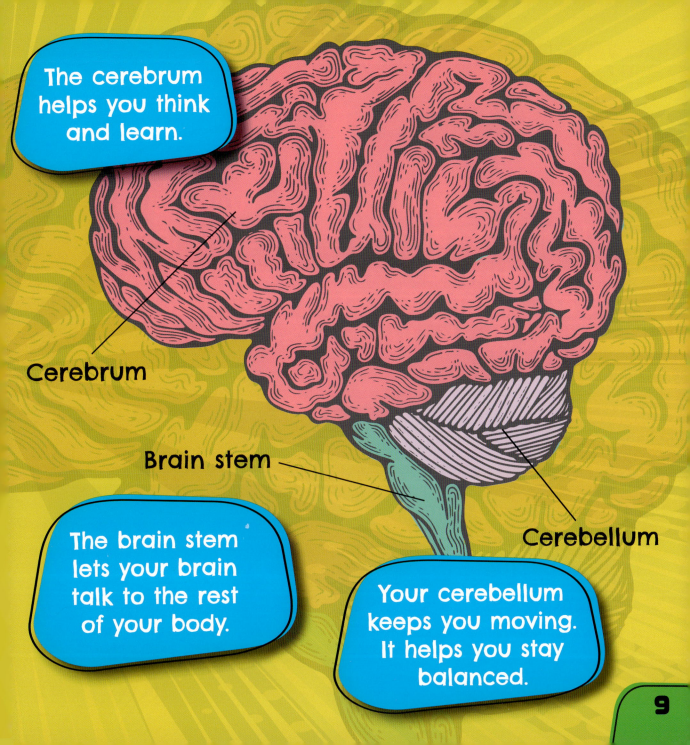

TALENTED TWINS

Your cerebrum has two twin sides. They are called the right and left **hemispheres** (HEM-i-sfeers). Each hemisphere has four **lobes**. What do the little lobes do?

Your left hemisphere controls the right side of your body.

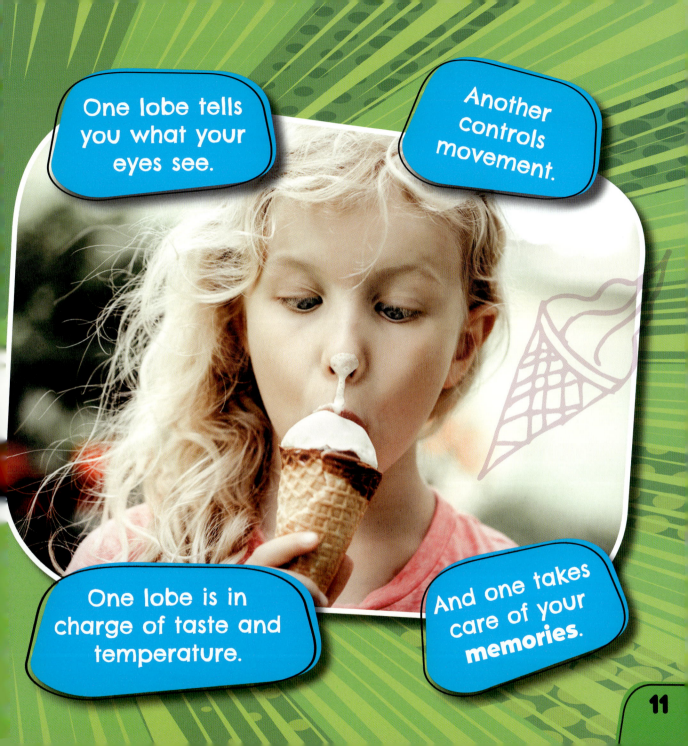

TAKING IT ALL IN

Your brain learns about the world around you. Then, your brain tells your body to act!

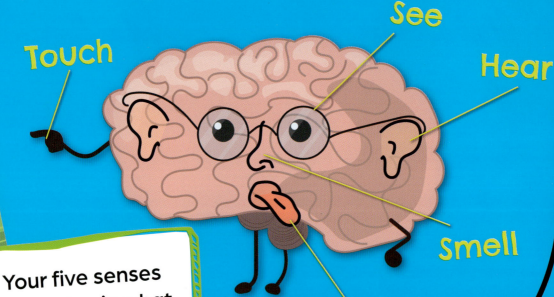

Touch
See
Hear
Smell
Taste

Your five senses tell the brain what is happening.

Sometimes, you *know* you think about the things you do. You tell your foot to kick a soccer ball. Other times, your brain works on its own! Your brain tells your body to breathe even when you aren't thinking about it.

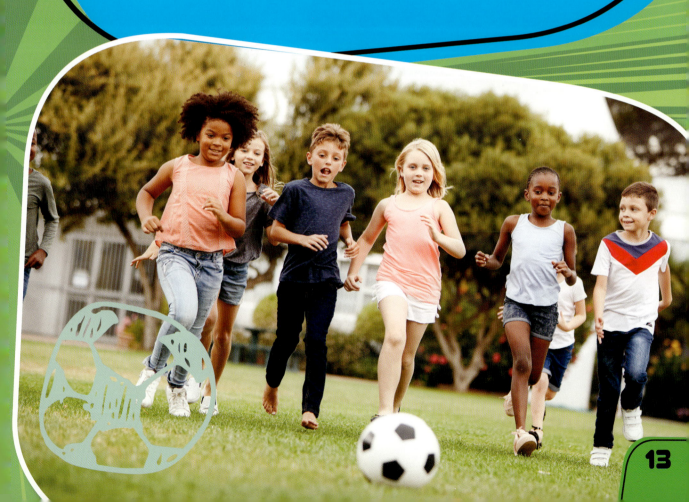

BRAIN BUDDIES

Your brain sends **signals** to your body, but it can't do it alone! The brain stem connects your brain to your **spinal cord**. This is the main highway between your brain and your body.

My messages travel through electricity inside your body.

14

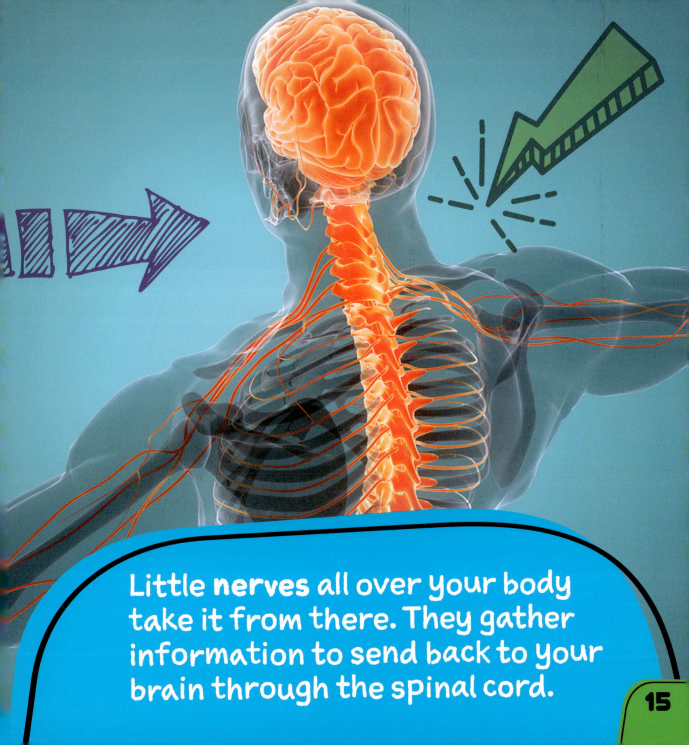

Little **nerves** all over your body take it from there. They gather information to send back to your brain through the spinal cord.

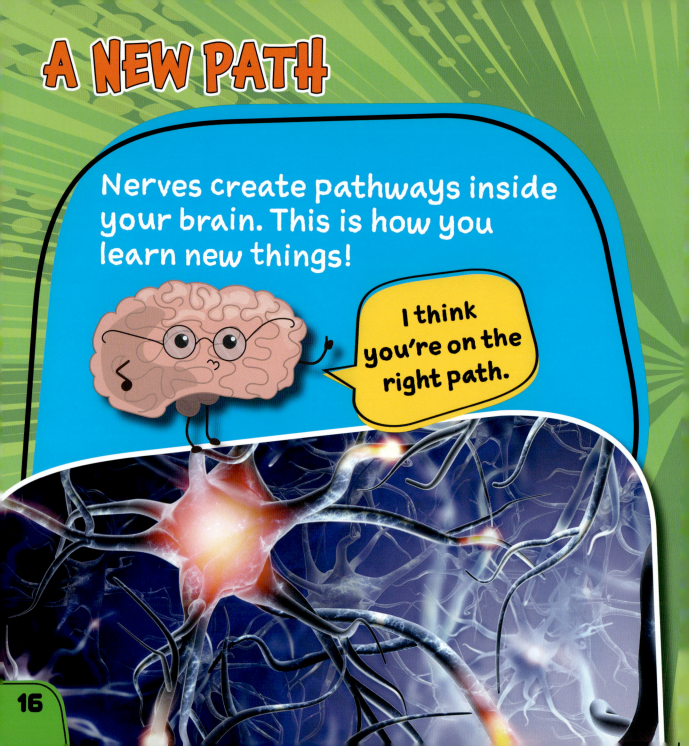

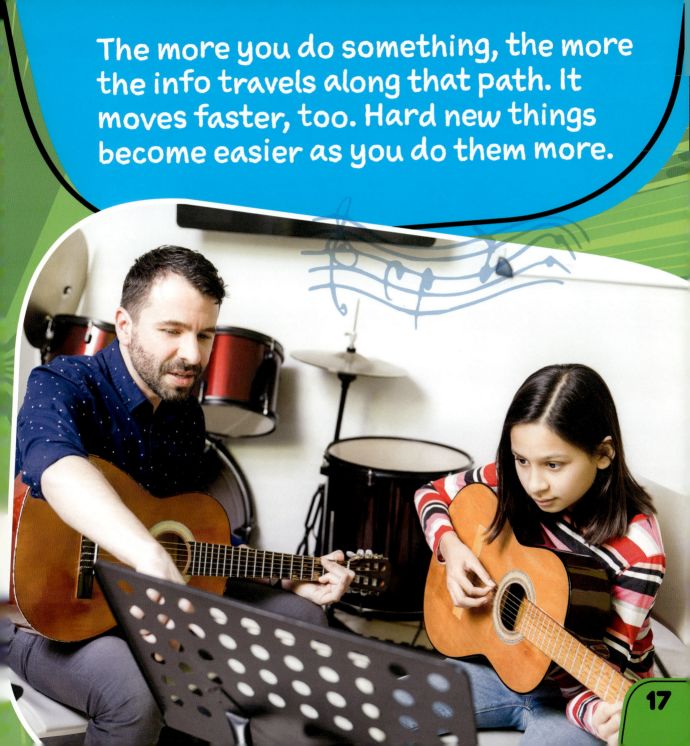

The more you do something, the more the info travels along that path. It moves faster, too. Hard new things become easier as you do them more.

TAKING CARE OF YOU!

When you take care of your brain, it takes care of you! Exercise sends blood to your brain. That's a good thing!

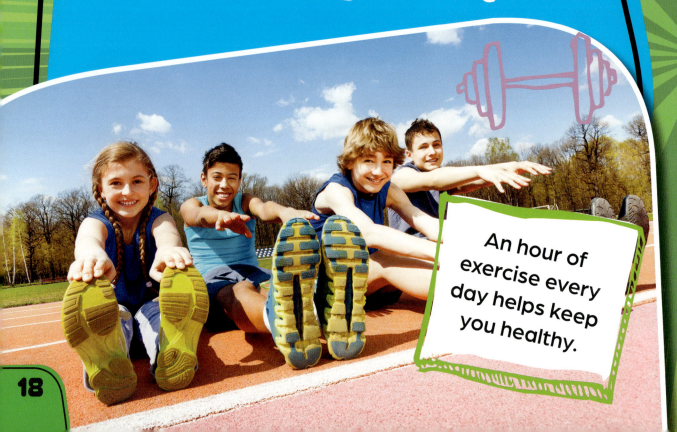

An hour of exercise every day helps keep you healthy.

Your brain needs **energy** to do its job! Eating well helps your brain do its best work. Foods like vegetables, fruits, and nuts are great for your brain.

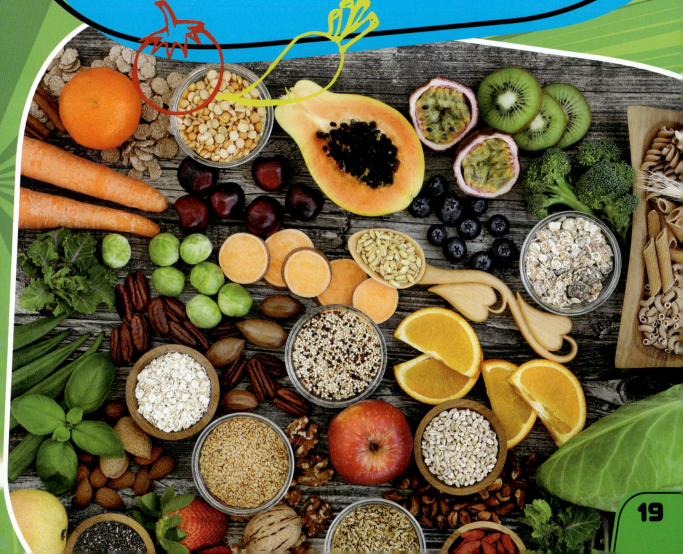

19

A GOOD NIGHT'S REST

Sleeping also helps your brain stay in tip-top shape. While you sleep, your brain is still hard at work.

Try to sleep for 9 to 12 hours each night.

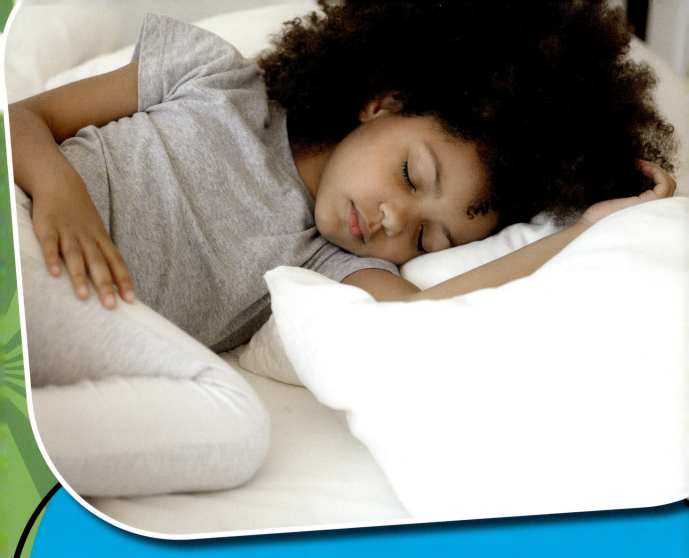

That's when your brain cleans up. It stores new info away for later in its memory. Do you remember anything that happened a long time ago? Thank sleep!

21

YOUR BUSY BODY

Your brain is an important part of the super machine that is your body. It works with lots of other things inside you. Together, they keep you going every day!

Taking care of your brain is a smart thing to do!

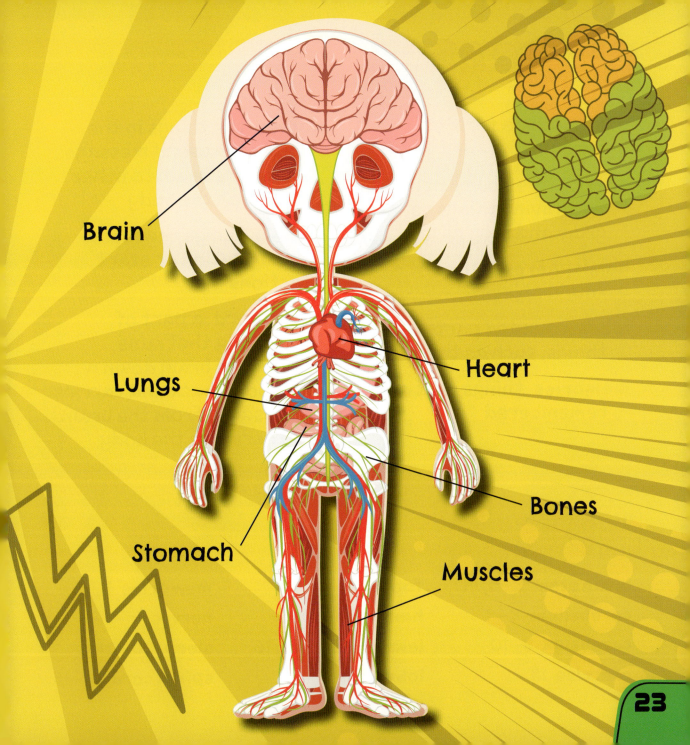

GLOSSARY

electricity a form of energy

energy the power needed by all living things to grow and stay alive

hemispheres halves of a round object

lobes rounded parts of things, such as the brain

memories things that are remembered

nerves the things in the body that send messages from the brain to other parts of the body

signals things that send information or start actions

spinal cord a part of the body that runs from the brain down a person's back and carries messages from the brain to nerves in the body

INDEX

brain stem 8–9, 14
cerebellum 8–9
cerebrum 8–10
exercise 18

food 19
hemispheres 10
learn 4–5, 9, 12, 16
lobes 10–11

memories 11, 21
nerves 15–16
sleep 20–21
spinal cord 14–15